This book is dedicated to
Chris Smith
L.P

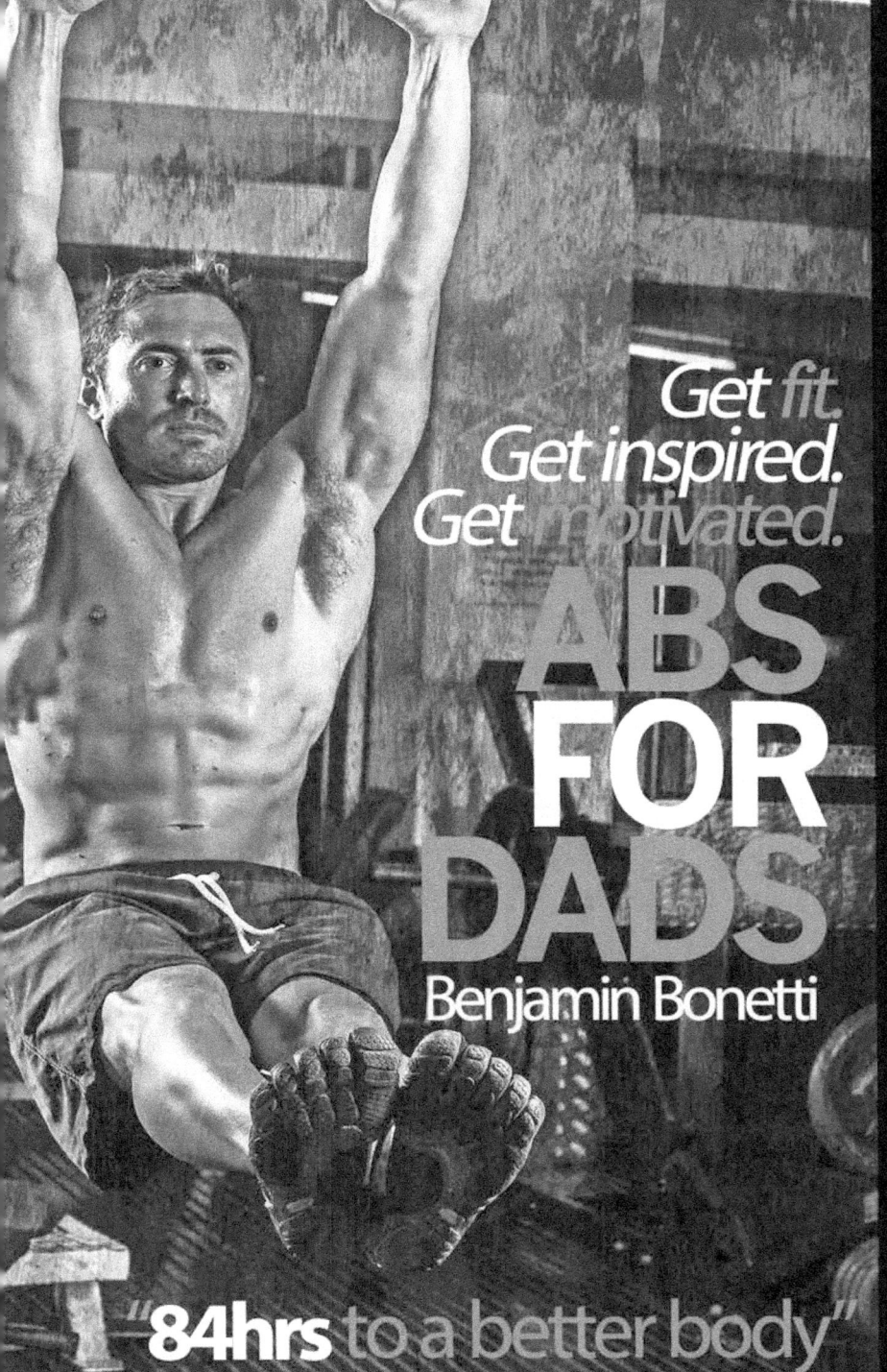

Get *fit.*
Get *inspired.*
Get *motivated.*

ABS
FOR
DADS

Benjamin Bonetti

"**84hrs** to a better body"

Contents

Foreword   **1**

Part One - The Boring Bits   **5**
Hard Fact 1   8
Hard Fact 2   11
Hard Fact 3   13
Hard Fact 4   17

Part Two - Nutrition Diary   **41**
Week 1   41
Weeks 2-6   42
Weeks 7-8   43
Weeks 9-12   43
Photoshoot Week   44
Extras   44

Part Three - Training Schedule   **47**
Monday   48
Tuesday   49
Wednesday   49
Thursday   50
Friday   50
Cardio Week One   50
Cardio Weeks Two - Five   51
Cardio Weeks Six - Eight   52
Cardio Weeks Nine - Twelve   53

About Benjamin Bonetti   **61**

If I can do it then so can you....

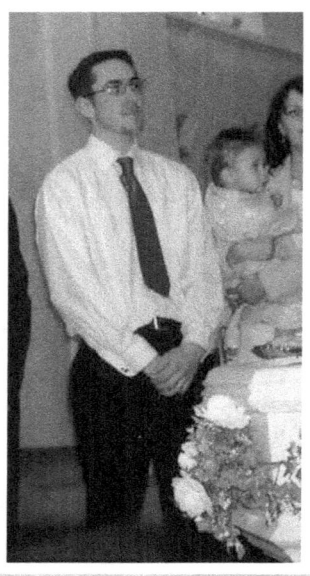

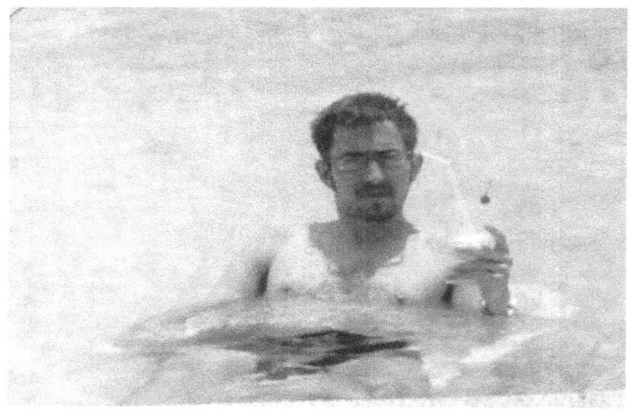

Foreword

I wasn't born with a six pack.

I am a father of two and a self-help author and I lead a relatively normal lifestyle. My job consists of inspiration, research and development, and mostly sitting on my behind staring at a computer screen. My diet has always been healthy, but I equally enjoy a pint or two, several bottles of red on occasion, and a take-away every now and then. A fairly standard lifestyle by modern standards I'd say.

I have always had an interest in sport, but I was the kid at school that wasn't picked for any team sports and I was usually left at the side-line or placed as a reserve instead. You know the one – the skinny kid. This all changed when I joined the army and the so-called three square meals a day began to boost my growth. My athletic ability peaked later than most, and, although I wasn't upper body strong, my distance running finally made me a popular choice among my peers.

When I left the army, my fitness went to pot. This was simply because it was my belief that I couldn't afford to eat the right foods or join a gym and my weight dropped off as a consequence. In fact, at one point, I would consider myself to have been border-line **very** underweight. Why?

Stress and attempting to raise a young family on a limited income were partially to blame, but education was 100 per cent the larger factor. It was my belief that "magazine models" were super humans who spent their life in the gym, injected every steroid possible, and had nutrition plans developed for them by crazy scientists wearing white coats and lab testing everything on animals...yes, that extreme, if not further crazed. Even further from the truth was my belief that the cost of eating the right foods exceeded my budget.

So with this belief structure, I, like most people, looked for an excuse. My ectomorph body type was by far the easiest factor to blame; **it** was the reason why I couldn't put on weight and the main argument I used when friends and family mentioned how slim/skinny I looked. There are a couple of pictures I will share with you which serve to demonstrate how small I actually got. The first was taken at my son's baptism, the second while I was on my honeymoon in the Maldives. Here you can see what I mean.

So, over the last 10 years, I have tried most of the available natural weight gain methods in an attempt to not only gain weight but also gain muscle. None of them worked. However, in the interests of fairness, I must admit that I found most of them were either too difficult to follow or virtually impossible to stick to due to the unrealistic restraints and restrictions in place. Worse still, many of them fail to offer the exact requirements so the end results you're likely to gain are left very much open to interpretation.

At school, the skinny kid and the fat kid always face the same dilemmas.

The new eating diary contained within these pages demonstrates just how easily these limiting beliefs can be changed. I changed, and I believe the simple and easy to understand steps will make it possible for you to do the same. There's no medical jargon and no "fitness speak", just plain and simple English.

This programme is also unlike most other conventional workout and diet schedules in other ways. Quite often a programme will shock your system from day one but in this programme, the gradual changes work in line with the changes you will see in your body, and this provides the additional motivation you might need to overcome any issues you face as you progress from week to week.

I have found this to be a much better approach than having to work harder to continue getting the results you want the further you go into a programme to continue getting the results you want. As I see it, if you look good in week 8 without feeling you've been beaten up then you're much more likely to continue into week 12 ... well, that's the plan.

It's at this stage I want to point out that this new eating programme isn't hard; it isn't designed to trick you or push you to insanity, it's designed to fit in with your lifestyle and allow you to achieve through re-educating yourself in good, nutritionally-rich eating habits. Of course, the further you go the more the extreme the diet becomes, but, as already mentioned, you can choose to use only the first stage of meal planning throughout the whole term. However, the likelihood is that the visual and emotional changes you begin to experience will encourage you to take the bull by the horns and push yourself to achieve that better you. I have run this training programme with some very sceptical people and even they have found themselves continuing to follow through each stage to the end with ease.

I would also like to point out that this new eating diary _is exactly_ what I went through. Nothing has been amended, forged or altered and for this reason you may need to alter some of the exercises to suit your personal end goal. With that said, if you do choose to follow it exactly as planned, I can guarantee that you will see massive transformational results within 12 weeks.

Note: Remember that each of us is different and therefore no two people are guaranteed to experience exactly the same results within the same time frame. Some of you may achieve your goals faster than others who are following the same plan, but the choice of whether to continue beyond the scheduled 12 weeks to gain your dream outcome is, of course, ultimately yours.

Within the following pages, I have provided notes and bullet points to outline the very basic "need to know" information. It's my belief that less is definitely more in terms of usability and effectiveness, but you can always conduct your own research should you wish to further your knowledge and understanding. As already noted, this isn't a nutrition journal per se but a diary of the processes I have used and honed to achieve the results I wanted. It's designed to be interactive so, just as you would take a pen with you when working out your training schedule, treat it like a diary. Take it with you and write in it when you're training ... use it and abuse it. I still have a dog-eared, water-damaged copy of my own that I take with me to the gym, and while it may be pretty tatty, it still serves as a reminder of the daily programme and my overall progress.

You may find you need to refer to the book fairly often in the first few weeks, and that's fine. Work at your own pace and keep in mind that there's no rush. Yes, it's a 12 week plan, but never lose sight of the fact that you have a lifetime to enjoy the results. Adopting this attitude helps to eliminate any pressure you may be feeling (unless you happen to be training for a specific event or a photo shoot!) and this in turn helps you to get the best results. Feeling pressured will only drain your energy and restrict your thinking, thereby counteracting all of your efforts and limiting your potential to succeed.

Part One
The Boring Bit

Let's Get Started...

Okay, starting your journey is the easy part – well that's what most will say! Starting for me is often the hardest part, and that's because there's a tendency to build a number of visual restrictions internally which inevitably highlight the "harder" aspects of the programme.

To eliminate this, the best advice I can give is to start training only when you know you can commit. This means that if you have something like a wedding or a work function coming up and you feel there's a strong possibility that you'll be tempted away from the programme, then it would be better to re-think your timing. Although the programme has been designed to deliver results easily, it still will require a certain amount of effort on your behalf and there's no room for corner-cutting.

Be prepared to alienate yourself; after the first few weeks, you will realise that you have started a gym-eat-sleep routine in which, without stating the obvious, you will find that the gym and your training becomes more important than coffee in the morning on the way to work or an after work pint on a Friday. Because of this simple change, you may experience a little pressure from your friends and family, but this will change once they begin to see the results you have achieved. In fact, you may even notice that more and more begin to contact you outside of the usual meeting points because they want to join you.

The standards you set are yours, so take ownership.

Of course, if you do feel pressured by resistance from friends and family, you can always come up with a one-liner to explain your reasons for doing what you're doing (not that you should have to) in a way that it's hard for them to respond negatively to. My one liner was:

"Well, I am the wrong side of thirty and I noticed my body had gone through some serious changes; I have got to do something about it, wouldn't you agree?"

Putting it this way makes it hard for them not to agree with you, especially if they are carrying a little extra weight themselves. However, it's always best to avoid these types of conversations, particularly if weight loss is a touchy subject, and just remember that not everyone wants to improve ... just because you are taking the action needed to become a better you doesn't mean that everyone else shares your ambition.

So, you have set the time, and you know you're likely to meet some resistance. Now what ...?

Understanding the bigger basic picture – that's what! You will hear, just as I have done, about many hundreds of different ways to lose weight, lose fat, gain muscle...it's not called the diet and fitness *industry* for nothing ... and it would seem that everyone and their dog has an opinion on how best to do it. But, as I have already pointed out, we are all different and there's no one-size-fits-all programme that will bring about exactly the same results in the same timeframe for every individual. There are those that will bring about permanent change with lasting results and those that will bring about immediate results but with limited long-term change. If you haven't guessed it already, the concept of this programme is to show you a better and more attractive way to achieve a baseline from which you can then go on to improve upon at your own leisure.

Of course, with so many opinions floating about out there, it should come as no surprise that there are a good few myths among them. You will no doubt have heard many of them or read about them in glossy "celebrity" magazines, but there are certain ones that absolutely must be "busted" if you want to make the most of your efforts. For example:

Myth

The "All-You-Can-Eat" Diet

Eat, eat, eat...eat as much as you want and eat whatever you want. Stop! Much as we might like the sound of this idea, if losing weight is your goal then eating as much as you want and whatever you want is NOT going to help you achieve it. *Exactly* the same is true if you want to gain muscle. I was told by many industry professionals that adding muscle was simply a case of eating truckloads of food and lifting progressively heavier weights. Not so! They said, "It doesn't matter what you eat, just eat it; eat, eat, eat some more, and *then* cut." It would seem to be common practice among many "bodybuilders" to bulk up with food as well as training before cutting back to reveal the muscle that has been hidden under a layer of flab. This is NOT a healthy practice.

Fact

The "My-Body-Is-A-Temple" Diet

It *does* matter what you eat. In fact, it matters considerably, and anyone who tells you otherwise needs to talk to an athlete who has achieved anything worth talking about ... although, having said that, this isn't necessarily true either when you consider the TV adverts that aired during the 2012 Olympics in which our medal winners promoted a certain fast-food restaurant!

Clearly, you can't always take it from the pros as they may well have "sold out" to capitalise on their own success, so take it from me instead: take it from me and the 10 years it has taken me to build a functional programme that works around the average lifestyle.

Fast food is for fatties, it is NOT for you ... use this affirmation next time you're considering a cream cake at your local bakers.

Fat and muscle are two completely different substances. Fat, once consumed, will always remain fat, and muscle will always remain muscle. Fat cannot turn to muscle and muscle cannot turn to fat, so anyone advising you to bulk up (in terms of trying to put on muscle) by eating fat should be ignored.

In terms of trying to shed unwanted weight, if you're going to be shedding pounds of fat, then cutting the amount of fat you eat and increasing the amount of exercise you do is the way to do it. However, in terms of both diet and exercise, it's not just about *quantity,* it's also about *quality.*

"If more goes in than comes out then you have an issue."

Hard Fact # 1: if you want to eat crap then expect to look crap, it really is that simple!

I have gained over 3 stone since my wedding day – that's 48 pounds of muscle, not fat – and I've gone from weighing just over 9 stone to 13 stone. Yes, it has taken time, but the time it has taken has included years of research, trial and error and learning the hard way what works and what doesn't as well as what to believe and what to ignore.

Does it really work or is it just another fad programme?

I know what you're thinking:

How can it work in just 12 weeks?

Are those photos for real?

Did the transformation really only take 12 weeks, or did it actually take much longer?

Yes, the transformation did take just 12 weeks and, yes, the photos are real! As I mentioned earlier, nothing has been left out. The photos haven't been edited in any way other than ensuring they fit in with the design of the book, and the food plan provided is gram for gram exactly the plan I followed. Complete transparency.

Is it going to work for you?

Well, that depends on how much you want to commit and how certain you are that you can do/follow what's asked of you. If you can, then it's guaranteed to work for you, if you can't, then please don't start as I wouldn't want this programme to join the many thousands of others that get added to the "failure" list or list of world's worst diets ...

... This is not a diet, it is a lifestyle choice, so please don't call it one.

It goes without saying that the food diary can only work if you follow it. If you don't, then it won't – simple! If you think you can sort of commit, or half commit, or you can commit to following it to a degree while throwing in a few extras, then, once again, please don't start. If you start it with this sort of attitude then you will only be wasting your time, effort and money ... and, more importantly, my reputation.

Why did I write it?

I have written and chosen to share my programme with others partly because I have an interest in the sporting and health arena, but mainly because of the radical changes I have experienced personally. Remember, I was the skinny kid at school. The physical *and* psychological changes I have achieved for myself are changes that everyone should be given the opportunity to experience. So many people fail to achieve their health and fitness goals because they believe, as I once did, that it's impossible to fit "training" into work and family life, or it's impossible to eat well on a limited budget. In writing this programme, it's my aim to dispel those mythical and limiting beliefs once and for all.

In the process of going through my own transformation, gym instructors, yes, that's right, professionally trained gym instructors at my "large commercial gym" often asked me what programme I was on. Rather than handing over my training diary, I decided that if they, the professionals, were going to offer it to their clients as an effective plan, then I shouldn't stop there but share everything I had learned with others who wanted to experience the same end results.

On the subject of gyms, in the time I've spent in commercially run gyms over the last few years, one thing has become apparent – they do not work. They work in a business sense, but they do not work in the interest of those looking to lose body fat (unless they are following a specific programme). For example, I see the same people at my gym smashing out 40 minutes on the cross trainer, step machine, running machine or bike every single day for months on end and yet it makes very little difference, if any, to their body shape. The next time you are at the gym, take a moment to notice the people around you; what are they doing? Chances are you're going to notice certain patterns of behaviour, but you'll also begin to notice that it's not just the time you spend in the gym that gets you results, it's what you *do* when you're in there! When you commit to the following programme, you're very quickly going to discover that it's not the person who spends most time in the gym who makes the greatest gains.

So here it is...

... A complete breakdown of cardio, weights and nutrition:

The only aspect I have left out is lifestyle, but this is easy to explain. I am currently writing two books, this one and another. This means I sit in front of a computer for about six or seven hours a day and I don't move much unless to stretch, let the dogs out, go to the toilet or eat – not forgetting visits to the gym. I'm married, have two children and two dogs, and a number of other hobbies, not least a keen interest in wildlife conservation which sees me studying for several hours a week in the evenings. I also have a couple of other business interests which take up some additional time each week: I have a mortgage and bills to pay and a large family that I like to see as much as possible, so, as you can see, I have a lifestyle that isn't particularly different to any other dad, and certainly no less busy – even before fitting in time to spend at the gym.

I make time ... it's simple; if I want results, I go and get them.

I mention this now because the most common excuse I hear used by people in the gym is, "I wish I had the amount of time you have," or, "I just don't have the amount of time in the evenings to prepare my meals in advance like you do." Well, let's just bust the unless-you-are-a-professional-athlete-it-is-impossible-to-find-time-to-eat-healthily-and-exercise-regulary myth right away, shall we? Listed below are the average amounts of time I spend in the gym and preparing food.

☐ **Gym Time** – no more than 60 minutes
☐ **Food Preparation Time** – 15 to 30 minutes

Now, when you consider the known fact that most people spend at least 55 minutes per day watching TV, surfing the net, or looking through social media websites, it becomes clear that time management is a much bigger issue than a lack of time.

Hard Fact # 2: we can all find time when it's something we want

to do, right?

If you can't go to the gym because you leave home for work too early in the morning, then look at going during your lunch break. If you can't manage at lunch, then look at going after work. If you need to get home straight after work, then look at going later in the evening. Most commercial gyms are open from 6.30am till 10.00pm, surely that's a big enough time window for anyone to commit just one hour.

Time isn't an issue ... so please don't make it your excuse. You *can* find an hour to spend at the gym, and you *can* find 15 minutes to prepare six meals in advance. If you're honest with yourself, you'll accept that 15 minutes of meal preparation time is probably less time than you currently need to prepare your meals.

What's next; and what's going to affect your progress?

Keep in mind that this is a diary and not a health nutrition book, and for this reason I've not gone into great detail on the sciences behind everything included. You may find that as your results begin to show and become clearer, you can refine things to suit your particular body type and tailor the details to create the exact end result you want. If you want to find out a little more by doing some research of your own, make sure you always look at both sides of every argument. For example, if one "expert" advises against eating a certain food, take the time to look into the flipside of the argument by reading what those who advocate the consumption of that food have to say. That way, you can form your own opinion of what's right for you based on your own beliefs and common sense.

That being said, there are the three things that I believe to be the largest contributing factors in terms of success when following this programme, regardless of any other opinions or previous studies.

1. Time – the amount of time you can commit; time for training, time for preparing and eating a healthy diet, and time for research if you choose.

2. Money – the amount of money you can comfortably invest in your wellbeing and nutrition.

3. Genetics – the way your body naturally responds to certain nutrients and stressors.

Note: Please do not assume that you have a medical condition until you have been tested via blood samples and have discussed the results with a health professional.

Hard Fact # 3: very few people actually *have* **medical issues** (so don't use them as excuses for gaining weight or lacking fitness!)

If you choose to look into alternative advice, keep the following in mind:

Medicine – medical opinions have changed over the years and many things we once believed to be true have now been proved false. Just as it was once a popular opinion that the world was flat, popular opinions in medicine are also subject to change through continuing education and scientific research. This means that if you're set on the use of medication, you should check with a reputable pharmacist regarding the latest advancements in the field of diet/training supplements rather than your GP, as they are more likely to be up to speed on the latest research findings.

Magic Pills – following on from the above, be very wary of "quick fixes"! The programme you're about to begin offers remarkable results in only 12 weeks, but it's important to realise that this programme is only the beginning of a new lifestyle, and the first 12 weeks of becoming a better, more energised you. Fitness cannot be stored, so it's never a simple case of dedicating 12 weeks to getting the results you want and then sitting back with nothing more to do.

Exactly the same can be said of pills, potions and tablets. There is no such thing as a quick, *permanent* fix, so avoid any magic pill that promises quick gains or losses. Anything claiming to generate rapid results will generally only be doing so through generating water loss – most of which will be the result of the caffeine content. This is *not* healthy, and it's certainly not a sustainable lifestyle option.

Fit Pros – many fitness professionals "repackage" existing information and offer it as something completely new. I call these people mixers; they take the facts and mix them in a way that appears different and revolutionary, but they are essentially just reinterpreting the same information that's available to everyone. Just be aware that a programme doesn't need to have "bells and whistles" to be effective!

Fit Fatties – there are individuals out there who offer advice that they really should be taking themselves! It's a sad fact that many of the health professionals offering patients advice on weight loss and healthy eating are actually overweight themselves. The same is true in many areas of the health and fitness industry. If a "gym-er" or fitness professional is promoting and pushing a particular product or service, it's my belief that they themselves should be a living advert for the benefits it brings. If they're not, I'd steer clear. The following programme is my programme, and the pictures I'm able to share with you as a result of following it are proof that I practice what I preach ... I don't just write about it.

This being said, you can make your own judgements on the advice given, just as you will with the details and advice given in this book. The books I recommend are by people who question "static" health advice, and as such are constantly pushing towards promoting a more health conscious society through making the "need to know" information easier to access and, most importantly, easier to understand. This is information we *all* need to know for the sake of our own health, and we should not be made to feel it's beyond our understanding.

What this book isn't ...

So, having covered the important aspects of what this book is about, let's take a moment to consider what this book isn't!

I can't promise that you are going to lose all of your unwanted body fat or that you're going to be the next Men's Fitness magazine front cover model within the next 12 weeks, but I can promise that you're going to see some amazing results – and at a healthy speed. By healthy, I mean that your body isn't going to go into shock, and you will continue to meet the demands of your Basal Metabolic Rate (BMR). Your BMR is simply the number of calories your body needs to fuel your everyday bodily functions when at rest. This 12-week programme is not a crash "diet" or an extreme training regime in any other way, it's designed to stimulate muscle growth and promote fat loss at a rate that's healthy and sustainable.

Be very wary of fitness books <u>guaranteeing</u> you that you'll be the next Daniel Craig!

Be prepared for a little stress. There can be no doubt that you will be groggy at times; you may suffer from headaches (especially when cutting your dairy) and, if you choose to opt for the "photo-shoot" aspect of the programme, then there's ever chance you're going to feel horrible! However, when you consider the overall effects of achieving *lasting* change, the initial unfamiliarity of it all is very easily overcome.

Something I can say for sure is that the feedback from "normal" people who have followed this programme is very positive. They are more than happy with the results; they have become self-motivated individuals who have reached their primary goals plus at least 10 per cent more just for good measure, and all without the need to have expensive gym mentors or personal trainers or the need to go for the more expensive eating option.

What else do you need to consider?

Let's get honest! Hard work and determination along with quality nutrition and advice is all that's needed to improve our lifestyle choices, but yet the majority of us deem it incredibly difficult to change, so why is this?

For example, have you tried a diet in the past and only completed the first stages before "giving up"; have you set out on a new fitness mission and bought all of the stuff only to stop within the first week, or have you set a New Year's resolution and given up by the first week of February?

Why?

My answer to this is very simple: we are told by the media and led to believe by the media that it's hard to change. As soon as you look at this diary, you will appreciate that it isn't hard at all. In fact, as my father said to me years ago, "Keep it simple stupid," and that's exactly what I've done. Of course, this is not because I believe you're stupid! By keeping things simple, I've made sure that the fundamental basics are clear and not open to interpretation. Red means red and black means black, there are no deviations and therefore there's no potential for confusion.

Common-sense prevails throughout this programme and, indeed, it should prevail in everything you do from this point forward. If you think something is bad or represents a bad choice for you, then the likelihood is that you're right. Trust your gut instinct.

So what's the spilt: is exercise the answer ... or is it about diet?

It is my belief that the following represents the most effective split:

☐ **80 % Diet** – what you eat influences your results much more than the amount of exercise you do! If you eat fatty foods, it doesn't matter how many weights you lift, you will never reach the goals you want.

☐ **15% Lifestyle** – if you are stressed at work, have a poor relationship, or have other stuff on your mind, you are unlikely to commit to the time needed and much more likely to give up when times get hard or the diet pushes you to the next level.

☐ **5% Fitness/Exercise** – although the smaller percentage, it has equal importance in terms of commitment. The more sessions you miss, the less likely it is you're going to achieve the results you want ... 12 weeks of commitment isn't asking for much when you consider the amount of time you have perhaps committed to doing nothing up until now!

Hard Fact # 4: It's no harder and no more complicated than eating less and doing more.

With the above in mind, let's get back to basics. Food is essentially your body's fuel source, providing the energy you need to perform, so if you feed it rubbish then that's exactly how you're going to feel. If, on the other hand, you feed it the best possible fuel you can, then you enter a whole new realm of awesomeness!

Remember that the limits, distances and exercises set out within this diary are exactly those I programmed my mind to work towards, but it's important that you should always work to your own limits. If you have specific goals, make it your aim to *always* work to that level and consistency. On the topic of consistency, wherever possible, ensure that you keep all processes exactly the same for at least the first 12 weeks. Once you have completed the first cycle, you can begin to add, substitute or take out certain aspects of the training, but in terms of getting the best possible results for your efforts, it's best to follow the first 12 weeks parrot fashion. By doing so, you will at least learn for sure what works for you and from this base of knowledge and understanding you're able to consider potential alternatives that might also work in your best interest. However, it's worth noting that several of my trusted guinea-pigs made no alterations to their programme at all once they'd completed the first 12 weeks, other than the addition of freedom when socialising.

In summary, this 12-week diary offers you a fantastic (even if I do say so myself) guideline to follow as you set yourself on course to achieving phenomenal success. Again, as already stated, the more you invest in it, the more you're going to see the results you want, and vice versa ... success breeds success. If you start, then ensure you finish, and, most importantly, do not start with the preconceived idea that this programme will not work for you – even if diets have failed to work for you in the past – because this one will.

Kit List

When I started out many years ago, I had a limited budget, so I appreciate that spending £500 on new kit or £100 per month on gym memberships perhaps isn't a viable option. However, there are some essentials that make all the difference in terms of comfort, thereby easing any pressures and making the journey more enjoyable.

☐ **Gyms** – start within your budget and consider all of the factors. Look at every facility an establishment offers and work out what it would cost to pay for each of them separately. You may find that a gym with every facility, and therefore a larger monthly fee, actually works out cheaper as an overall package. Travel expenses must also be considered; a lower monthly fee doesn't represent good value if it costs you more to get there each time. Of course, if you have a home gym that fulfils the role, then this can work equally well.

☐ **Training Attire** – start with what you have, as it is likely that it will not fit soon! Look to change your kit at week 4 when you will begin to see and feel visible changes in your body shape, whether it's fat loss or muscle gain. Training kit for the gym doesn't need to be expensive, and you can often pick up some really good deals by looking at the "offers" section of fitness website pages. My advice is to simply buy the best you can afford, and keep in mind that lightweight materials are a much better bet than heavy cottons or wools which only retain heat and sweat.

☐ **Shoes** – aim for the best you can buy from day one. My father gave me a great piece of advice several years ago when he said, *"Buy a good pair of shoes and a good bed; if you are not in one, you are in the other."* For me, training shoes are an area in which the budget cannot be cut. Get your feet measured, and then look online for the best prices in that size. Bear in mind that each shoe manufacturer produces footwear to their own "standard" sizes, meaning a size 9 in one brand might be slightly bigger or smaller in another. Ideally, get shoes that are suitable for general gym work and for any outside cardio you may do, and if you need advice, visit a fitness shop that specialises in footwear. Always buy your footwear from someone who clearly has a strong interest in fitness and an understanding of your needs, and be clear about your budget as well as your intended use. It's no good having the best-looking pair of shoes in the shop if they're not designed for your purposes.

☐ **Gloves** – so many people avoid using gloves in the gym because they feel it's less manly! I personally use them because they protect my fingers and hands from becoming callused. I can recommend a product known as ProGripsTM, as I find they offer a good alternative to gloves and they're much easier to slip on and off whenever they're needed.

☐ **Water Bottle** – there are many different types of water bottle on the market, each offering a credible design. Personally, I prefer one that incorporates a filter, simply because I believe it eliminates any potential for contamination from gym water supplies or any refill points.

☐ **Tupperware Pots** – you will need 8 pots (or more if you want) for your meal planning. You can pick these up from anywhere but it's a good idea to keep them all the same if possible. I have 6 identical pots with MEAL 1-6 clearly labelled on the lid. This not only keeps things simple, it also reduces the risk of picking up the wrong meal if I'm ever heading out of the door in a rush.

☐ **Liquidiser/ Juicer** – I only recently upgraded my liquidisers but it's possible to pick up a perfectly adequate machine for around £20 at most high street electrical goods stores. I use them to make smoothies and to mix protein shakes to my preferred consistency, but I actually prefer liquidisers over juicers as they retain 100 per cent of the ingredients. Of course, if you don't like "bits" in your drinks, then a juicer might be the best option for you.

☐ **Cash & Carry Card** – you can significantly reduce your monthly spend on meat by shopping at your local cash and carry. Some are restricted to business owners only, so do some research to find the ones that are open to the public in your area. Depending on where you live, you might also find some good online suppliers who will deliver directly to your door.

☐ **Music Player and Headphones** – if you do not have a training partner, there's nothing better than sticking on some tunes and getting in the zone! Most modern phones have a built in mp3 player so utilise this if you can, and I have found the best headphones to be the in-ear variety, however this is a personal choice.

☐ **Training Diary** – your training diary and a pen are, of course, the most important bit. This simple to use tool should be on hand at all times so that you can refer to it and take instruction. Remember to use it and abuse it; the more you add notes, the more you can refer back to it at a later date and use the information to gain a better understanding of what to improve on next time.

"Take care of your body. It's the only place you have to live."
- Jim Rohn

Sleep

The connection between sleep, muscle gain and fat loss is much greater than most think. Sleep can increase your motivation or not; it can aid your recovery or not, and it will either enhance your lifestyle or – you guessed it – not.

In order to maximise your results, you need to work on the basis of achieving at least 9 hours of sleep per night. I appreciate that this number of hours is higher than most other recommendations, but it's a number that I personally deem to be a suitable amount. Plus, if you aim for 9 hours and then miss out on a couple of those through the week, you will still have met the quota recommended by the majority of medical professionals.

If you have not been a big sleeper before now, perhaps feeling that it's a waste of your day, and you cannot bring yourself to begin sleeping this amount of time or you simply can't, then my advice is to listen to some audiobooks while lying in bed. Have a look at some of the nutritional, fitness or motivational podcasts available, or perhaps find an audiobook related to your specific hobby. Either way, get into bed and use this time to relax.

"The individual who says it is not possible should move out of the way of those doing it." Anon

Enjoy Your Coffee Fix (Caffeine)

I love coffee. In fact, since I began doing some hard-core research for this book over the last several months, I have become quite the coffee connoisseur. The whole process intrigues me; from the way it is developed to how it has been adapted and morphed to become the "instant" crap most people drink today.

Coffee is good, no matter what you think or how you feel. Caffeine has been proven many times over to improve health, both physically and mentally, and various studies have shown that it helps to prevent heart related illnesses, reduce the potential to suffer mental illness, and, in some instances, reduce the aging process. Of course, all of these findings relate to coffee consumption within reasonable limits. Common sense must always prevail ... and this applies to all of the advice given in this book.

I'd recommend spending just a few minutes this weekend researching coffee, its evolution and the health benefits ...

... Have a quality filter coffee before working out and feel the buzz!

Caveat: avoid drinking coffee after 6pm unless training, and then no later than 8pm.

> *"When it comes to eating right and exercising, there is no 'I'll start tomorrow.' Tomorrow is disease."*
> - V.L. Allinear

Get Creative With Your Food

During my time of trying out new things and being my own guinea-pig over the last several years, I have tasted some truly revolting so-called health kicks. One thing I learned early on is that diets (I hate this word but for ease of use I will use it here in a negative sense) need to be engaging otherwise they will fall apart and fail within the first few weeks of starting.

For a start, diets generally fail because they don't re-educate and they are simply unsustainable. They also tend to have a start and a finish, meaning that once you achieve the end result or the target weight you wanted, you then relapse into old habits straight away.

To avoid this, you need to get to know your foods and learn how to make them appetising. I have found the best way to do this is to get creative with spices. Spices are not only a great way to change the flavour of a meal, they also add a whole new dimension to the benefits of healthy eating. For example, turmeric's antioxidants help protect your cells from free radical damage. Antioxidants (contained within many natural spices) are also key nutrients in supporting your memory function, promoting your heart health, and boosting your immune system.

It's a fact that most households only vary their existing weekly diet from one week to the next by two or so items. This means that if you were to compare your shopping list from last week to this week then the food varieties and the planned meals are likely to be very similar, if not the same. Healthy eating is in fact a lot better, and a lot more interesting: there are more creative things you can do with a frying pan, a few spices and a chicken/turkey breast than a readymade meal!

Think about it for a moment; if you like curries then you can start making and creating your own recipes. With your eggs, you can make any number of omelette varieties using spices, chillies, nuts and dried fruits ... there are no limits in terms of creativity. And, if you ever get stuck for ideas, there are millions of online recipes that take just a few seconds to find.

Excite the mind with food.

One thing that any one of my friends and family will say about me is that I love my food. In my world, if food doesn't get you excited then something is going very wrong. This is something that worried me at first when designing and engineering the shopping list for this programme, but, as I have mentioned, the number of alternative meals and flavours you can create with your ingredients is more than you will be able to consume within the following 12 weeks. So, if you're like me and love food, you are really going to enjoy the mixture and the spice adventures. However, if you see food as simply an essential, then you can stick to the basics and only add a few spices when you want.

Tip: when talking about food and your new lifestyle eating habits, avoid the word DIET. In fact, avoid using any word with the word DIE in it.

"To keep the body in good health is a duty... otherwise we shall not be able to keep our mind strong and clear." - Buddha

IF – Intermittent Fasting

At times, for whatever reason, you may find yourself bored by the mere thought of facing another meal. If, for example, you find that just the thought of another chicken or turkey breast disgusts you, you can choose this day to fast. Although this is something I would recommend restricting to a maximum of 4 days over the whole 12 weeks, it does have its benefits and it sort of resets and motivates the mind to get back on track.

I only IF'd for 3 days within the whole period and each of those days was towards the end of the programme. Emotionally and mentally I was strong, but I just woke up one day and couldn't see myself enjoying those daily meals, so I simply kept the water intake high and still enjoyed my post workout shake.

Your body can deal with this small amount of fasting, and when looking back to the lifestyle of our ancestors, food wouldn't always have been scheduled at regular intervals anyway due to the precariousness of availability and supply. So, if times get tough then take a day off. However, remember to keep the liquids coming.

"A bear, however hard he tries, grows tubby without exercise."
- A.A. Milne, Winnie-the-Pooh

Feeding/Fuelling

If you haven't noticed already from flicking ahead to take a peek at the meal planning, you will notice that it seems to include a lot of food. This "feeding to diet" concept has been used for many years within the bodybuilding industry and although some consider it outdated and unnecessary, I have found that it works well, especially when committing to gym training and lifestyle changes.

If you look at the meal timings, you will notice that throughout the day there is never more than a three hour gap between meals, meaning it's very unlikely that you will ever become hungry, and, if you do, it's only a short while before you can replenish.

Why eat so often?

The concept of eating frequently is very simple. By eating more often, your body spends more energy digesting the food thus speeding up the metabolism. You can go deeper into the science behind it with your own research, but that's the very basics of it. As you are eating clean (low fat), your body, after a period of adjustment, will begin to use its reserves, and this leads to a reduction in body fat.

"A man's health can be judged by which he takes two at a time –
pills or stairs."
- Joan Welsh

Cost Of Food

If you are worried about the cost of meat (protein), then remember that significant savings can be made by sourcing a local Cash and Carry, or by talking to your local butcher/farmer. When I first trialled this programme, I was amazed at the cost of the meat – around £100.00 per week from the local superstore deli counter at the time. Thinking this was a little excessive, I went to my local Cash and Carry butchery department, and here it worked out at around £25.00 per week for the same amount, the only difference being that it wasn't cut to specific weight. Please note that the meat I buy is *fresh* meat, not frozen, and it's important to realise that many frozen meats are filled / soaked to bulk up the weight of the product. Fresh is best.

With the meat sorted, it's now time to talk about the vegetables. I prefer frozen vegetables simply because I feel they last longer, and the nutrition is locked in earlier, especially with "frozen at source" varieties. The same applies to the fruit you will be using in your shakes. I find frozen fruits to be much more convenient and there's also less wastage.

Caveat: if you have a relatively unlimited budget then buy fresh from your local farmers market. They offer meat and vegetables that are picked and displayed within days, you can trace the location and source, and you need only buy the amount you need to see you through to the next market visit.

Weekly Spending

☐ **Budget:** £50 or less
☐ **High End:** £200 or more

What about vegetarians?

There are many vegetarian options to replace the meat (protein) choices, so it comes down to personal choice. Vegetarian sources of protein include beans and legumes, nuts and seeds, tempeh, tofu, soybeans and seitan.

> *"Those who think they have not time for bodily exercise will sooner or later have to find time for illness."*
> - Edward Stanley

Stay Clear Of Scales

People using their weight on the scales as a means of tracking and declaring their progress is one of my pet hates. Yes, I know this goes against nearly all other fitness training and weight/fat loss programmes available but the idea with this programme is to avoid getting sucked into the daily cycle of feeling deflated whenever the scales haven't changed. In fact, the needle on my scales hardly moved throughout the whole 12-week programme, but, clearly, my body shape changed. So how can this be? Well, it's simply because I lost the weight of body fat and gained the weight of muscle. The idea isn't to shed loads of weight, but to work towards creating a healthy ratio between body fat and lean mass. Along with every pound of fat lost, there should be a corresponding gain in muscle. Of course, this isn't always possible and it must be realised that if you're carrying an excessive amount fat then this ratio will vary.

Instead of using scales, the best form of measurement is the eye. If you look in the mirror and you can see a visual difference, then you've got all you need to gauge every inch of progress! From this point forward, make it a weekly routine to take a photo every Monday. It can be a full body shot or just the upper half, but the idea is to create a visual diary of the changes in your body shape as they happen. It might seem that there's very little difference in the first few weeks but when you look back over the photos after completing the first cycle, you will certainly notice the variants and where and when each change took place.

If you are dead-set on measuring the actual amounts of weight lost, then my advice is to use a set of body fat callipers. If you are a member of a gym, a free body fat analysis is generally part of the package but you can buy your own set on eBay for less than a few pounds. There are a number of online resources available to help you work out how to use them and make accurate calculations, however, if you choose the DIY approach it's important once again not to get sucked into taking measurements too frequently. Bi-weekly is often enough as it's unlikely that there will be any significant difference in the readings if taken any more frequently.

Another measuring tool that's likely to bring about the most enjoyment, and prove to you that the programme is working effectively, is the difference you begin to feel in your clothes. As you are now aware, you may not lose weight but your body shape and dimensions will change. For example, I can no longer fit into a pair of my favourite skinny jeans. This is because my quads have grown and I am unable to sit down comfortably when wearing them, yet my waist is still about the same size.

I know you will be tempted to reach for the scales, but resist. If needs be, remove them from your house all together until the 12 weeks are up. The true gauge of how well you have done isn't in those little numbers that show on the scales, but in the euphoric feeling you experience when you look in the mirror and like what you see.

> *"A fit, healthy body—that is the best fashion statement"*
> - Jess C. Scott

Daily Chocolate Fix

Yes, that's right, you *can* enjoy chocolate for the first 11 weeks of the programme by having 1 cube (not a bar) of dark chocolate every day. I preferred to stick to fair trade 80 per cent dark chocolate but most other varieties of plain chocolate will do. You can have this at any time throughout the day, the choice is yours, but through a process of trial-and-error I found the best time for me was just after my second to last feed at around 6pm.

Why dark chocolate?

Dark chocolate consumption (in moderation) has many known benefits. Listed below are just a few:

☐ Dark chocolate improves blood flow and may help prevent the

28

formation of blood clots. Eating dark chocolate may also prevent arteriosclerosis.

☐ Dark chocolate increases blood flow to the brain as well as to the heart, so it can help improve cognitive function.

☐ Dark chocolate also contains several chemical compounds that have a positive effect on your mood and cognitive health.

☐ Dark chocolate is loaded with antioxidants. Antioxidants help free your body of free radicals which cause oxidative damage to cells.

If you feel like experimenting with your daily allowance, try grating it over a prepared shake or even your coffee. Remember, it's your sanity kick, so use it in a way that's going to bring you the most enjoyment!

Tip: my favourite was to break it up into small pieces and add it to a bowl of mixed nuts and dried chillies.

"Health is the greatest of all possessions; a pale cobbler is better than a sick king."
- Isaac Bickerstaff

During / Post Training Nutrition

Millions of supplements suppliers would have you believe that their latest product is an absolute must if you want to maximise your training efforts and replenish your natural resources. The truth is that the only source of hydration you need is water – pure and simple. Bottled water is the best choice as it contains all of the essential minerals, but when this isn't an option, filtered tap water is the next best thing. Obviously, buying a bottle of water every time you need a drink can become prohibitively expensive but, once again, buying in bulk from the Cash and Carry is a great way to bring costs down.

Avoid ALL sugary drinks and any kind of stimulant or supplement during your session as you simply don't need them. In fact, they are likely to hinder rather than help your progress, so save your money and put it towards buying some new training kit when you reach week 4 instead.

Sugar serves no nutritional value while training.

Post training is a very different story. Again, just keeping things simple, I would opt for a quality nutritional product which is high in protein and low in fats and carbs. I experimented with a variety of the products available and my personal recommendation is offered at a discount at the rear of the book. It all comes down to personal choice but this particular combination worked best for me.

"When health is absent, wisdom cannot reveal itself, art cannot become manifest, strength cannot be exerted, wealth is useless, and reason is powerless."
- Herophiles

Supplements

Okay, supplementation is a very topical subject and if you have done any form of training previously then you will probably already have your own preferences. However, it's my personal belief that very few of the products on the market actually provide any of the benefits promoted on their labels.

I will base my recommendation on what I have used and what works – nothing more, nothing less. There are plenty of people who will advise you otherwise, but, for me, I can only base my knowledge on the extensive research I have completed and my own human guinea-pig trial.

☐ **Whey Protein** - whey protein is regarded as a supplement staple, used by athletes, bodybuilders and fitness enthusiasts to help with muscle recovery, lean muscle growth, and general health.

☐ **BCAA** – the BCAAs are among the nine essential amino acids for humans, accounting for 35 per cent of the essential amino acids in muscle proteins and 40 per cent of the preformed amino acids required by mammals.

☐ **Multivitamins** – a multivitamin is a preparation intended to be a dietary supplement with vitamins, dietary minerals, and other nutritional elements.

☐ **Omega Oils** – omega-3 fatty acids are a group of three fats called ALA, EPA, and DHA.

Although I would love to be able to say that you are going to get all of your essential nutrients from the natural foods included in your diet and therefore supplements are simply not required, it's very unlikely to be the case in reality as achieving the required daily dosage would mean eating a much larger quantity of food than required every day.

At the rear of the book, you will find a link to the products I have used. I trialled a great many, so I have included only those I actually used throughout the 12-week programme.

"A stationary bike is a device that epitomizes the phrase "hurry up and wait."
- Jarod Kintz

Technique

If you are lifting weights for the first time, or perhaps you've have been out of the game for a while, you must get a gym professional to show you how to do it properly. I see more people hurting themselves at the gym through poor technique than anything else and injuries like this are totally avoidable.

The use of correct technique is better for a number of reasons – not least injury prevention – but primarily it will allow you to lift heavier weights in a shorter period of time. I have seen smaller (muscular) individuals lift nearly twice the amount of larger individuals simply on the basis of technique. Nail it early on and you will reap the rewards of this programme a lot faster.

"Get comfortable with being uncomfortable!"
- Jillian Michaels

Weight Increments

The best advice I can provide is to start low. We all want to impress others in the gym with our max lifting ability but, in truth, correct form and technique is more important. Once you have mastered the correct form using lighter weights then you can begin to add weight progressively from there.

When I started, I used only the bars to master the correct technique and then added only the amount of weight I could lift without losing good form. Unbalanced form can cause injuries fast so *always form first*. Below is a practical guideline to the increments you should be looking to achieve. Keep the first few weeks comfortable before loading the weight, and ensure that you have someone to spot/ support you when completing max lifts.

☐ Up one weight (min 5kg) per fortnight on free-weights. For example; week 1 you are benching 40kg, week 4 you will bench 45kg, week 6 you will bench 50kg etc.

☐ Up one weight per fortnight on cable weights. For example; week 1 on the rope crunches you are using 27.5kg, the following increase you raise it to 32.5kg.

☐ The cardio is self-explanatory, but you do have the choice to increase or decrease the time/distance by 20 per cent from week 4. This is based on your own comfort zones and should be regulated to your own "true" ability.

Remember, you are using heavy weights that hurt when dropped on bodily parts! Keep your training within sensible boundaries to eliminate any chance of unnecessary injury.

"The reason fat men are good natured is they can neither fight nor run."
- Theodore Roosevelt

Injury

Due to the nature of the exercises, should you suffer an injury (although there is no reason that you should, so don't use a convenient "injury" as an excuse), seek medical attention as soon as possible. Avoid thinking that you will deal with it yourself, or that just taking a few days off will sort things out, speak to a medical professional and take their advice. Stop the training aspect of the programme until you have been given the all clear from your professional, but continue with the eating aspect of the programme at the same level.

When you are able to return to physical training, deduct two weeks from where you left off and resume as normal from that point. You may find that you recover quicker as the process continues and that you are equally motivated to get back into training. For example: if you become injured in week 3, stop physical training but continue with week 3 diet. If you are given the all clear a week later, return to week 1 of physical training and continue until both week 3 diet and training are back in sync.

Note: make sure you keep to the recommended full recovery period; if you hit the gym too early there's much greater potential to become injured again and cause further delays in your training as a consequence.

"No body is worth more than your body"

- Melody Carstairs

Positive & Negative Food Values

This is something I feel it's important to include; it's simple.

☐ A positive food value is something that when you look at it, you know it is going to add value to your training programme either in terms of sugar content, carbs or protein.

☐ A negative food value is the opposite. When you look at it, you know immediately that it is processed and contains chemicals that you're unable to even pronounce.

With every new food choice you make from this point forwards, ask yourself, "Is this going to positively benefit my body?"

"It's easier to stay in shape if you never let yourself get out of shape in the first place."
- Bill Loguidice

Reality Check

Okay, here's the harsh reality: it's important to remember that we are all individuals and for this reason, everyone begins this programme from a unique starting point. The different shapes and sizes at the start are inevitably going to create different end results, and your individual body shape is going to determine your final "look" and appearance. Keep the following in mind:

1. We are not all genetically as strong as one another, meaning that someone starting the same programme at the same time as you may achieve greater or lesser gains no matter how committed each of you remains. Based on this fact, it's important to set your own visual goal and not that of another.

2. It takes a large amount of determination to break the 4 week point. Basically, after 4 weeks of training and eating in accordance with this programme's nutritional diary, you should have broken the old, unhealthy habits. However, up until the 4-week point you are still open mentally to a relapse.

3. Accept that 99 per cent of the images you see in fitness magazines are airbrushed. When starting out on your fitness programme, you may flood your evening's reading with fitness related material, and there's no harm in doing so as it focuses your attention on the industry. However, be aware of falling into the trap of thinking that your personal results aren't as good as the individuals featured in the glossy pages. Many of the fitness professionals and athletes you will see have spent years mastering their training technique and they will usually have invested heavily in achieving their results.

4. Make sure you have the time to commit to changing your body. Although we would all like to take a pill and awaken with a great physique the following morning, it's not going to happen that way. However, committing to making positive changes to your diet and embarking on an effective physical training plan *will* bring you the results you want. As I have said before, it takes time to re-educate your body and mind into "thinking healthy" so make a 1 hour per day commitment for the next 12 weeks of this programme.

"If you don't do what's best for your body, your the one who comes up on the short end."
- Julius Erving

Shakes – Having Fun With A Blender

I love shakes, not the fatty readymade types but the ones you make yourself. There is something about throwing a load of ingredients into a pot, mixing them up, and then tasting your homemade concoction that's hard to beat – I think it's the creativity and the birth of the unknown.

Homemade blended adventures are a great addition to the usual training programme. Not only do they add a bit if excitement, they also bring an element of sanity to the mix. I have upgraded my blending basics recently but it doesn't need to be expensive to get started. All you need is a pot you can use for the ingredients and a blender.

You will also need three key elements. These are:

☐ Ice (not strictly required but I much prefer shakes with ice)
☐ Almond Milk /Soya Milk/ Water
☐ Flavour / Ingredients

The flavour/ingredients are essentially anything that you would consider a positive food value. However, there have been times during my cheat meal (see below) where I have blended cheesecake ... it was awesome and within my 1 hour!

Here are some of the sampled flavour/ingredients I used:

Kiwi, almonds, walnuts, spinach, apples, bananas, pineapple, melon, peach, plum, pear, orange, broccoli, chocolate, peanut butter, honey, shannon fruit, lychees, cucumber.

Check out my Facebook page for more blends.

> *"If your dog is fat, you're not getting enough exercise."*
> - Author Unknown

Get ready for head games...

Like anything new, there will be times when you will be asking yourself if it's all worthwhile and if you should carry on or jump to the next alternative programme. The first thing to understand is that this is perfectly normal. When faced with resistance, our bodies naturally want to rebound, just like an elastic band. Why? Because it's easy ... well, so your mind thinks. The truth is that it's actually harder.

The more you relapse, the more difficult it becomes to make changes. During this programme, you will be changing the way your body has "coped" with poor nutrition and lazy eating for however long before now. Your mind and body will have become used to dealing with certain chemicals and to doing its best to counteract them throughout this time, therefore it's going to take a little while to adapt. The more you relapse, the more you delay the process of change as your body slips into rebounding to avoid change ... and so the cycle continues.

During this adaptation process, be prepared for some serious head games. For example, when I removed dairy products from my diet, I experienced bad headaches for the first 8 days. But, from that point forwards, I can honestly say that my mental clarity has been improved by at least 10 per cent. Your body will respond differently to each step of the programme; just keep going and accept that this is completely normal. Everyone who follows this programme will experience some form of challenge at some point so remember that it's only resistance and you can push through it by keeping your head "in gear"!

"The difference between someone who is in shape, and someone who is not in shape, is the individual who is in shape works out even when they do not want to."
- Unknown

Visual Reminders

Having an image in your mind of the end result you're aiming for is a great way to keep your head in gear and motivate yourself to keep going. Actual visual reminders are also powerful motivators, both towards and away from certain outcomes. For example, I have a picture of myself when I weighed less than 9 stone and a magazine image of a fitness professional who I believe has a physique that will compliment my build. In these two images, I have a visual reminder of what I'm working away from and what I'm working towards.

Create a visual prompt that works for you. Be realistic – remember that not all magazine images feature *real* people – and put it where it will serve as a reminder on several occasions throughout your normal day. The fridge door is a good place because it's not only somewhere you visit on a regular basis, it also acts as a positive deterrent should you be thinking of opening the door to get yourself a little extra treat.

> *"Physical fitness can neither be achieved by wishful thinking nor outright purchase."*
> - Joseph Pilates

Cheat Meals

I have two thoughts on cheat meals:

1. If you are overweight, you've had plenty of cheat meals in the past and therefore you shouldn't have any now.

2. At times, it's just nice to indulge in something you know you shouldn't be.

To strike an acceptable balance between these two lines of thought, I have included one full hour in each month throughout the 12-week programme in which you can consume as much as you can/want. It's my personal experience that once you've allowed yourself to indulge in this way, you naturally tone down your indulgences next time around, and you're more than likely going to choose not to indulge at all.

It's a good idea to share the "cheat meal" experience with someone else, and it's best to prepare and diarise the planned hour so that you can simply start the clock and enjoy. Just to help you put things into context, I consumed oveßr 10 000 calories during my first hour of permitted indulgence!

Part Two
Nutrition Diary

This is the exciting part, and it has been divided into four sections. Each section has been developed to work in line with the physical training coming up in part three, and to gradually reduce your food intake.

Section 1 = Week 1
Section 2 = Weeks 2-6
Section 3 = Weeks 7-8
Section 4 = Weeks 9-12

Collate your shopping list at the rear of the book. The meals are to be consumed at 3 hour intervals and the first meal can be at whatever time you plan to have your breakfast. During my training, the first meal started at between 6am and 7.30am.

To make things simple, prepare your meals the evening before. The meal preparation process speeds up as you progress through the programme but it generally takes no more than 15 to 30 minutes in total.

Week 1

Meal 1 (breakfast): 5 egg whites + 1 yolk and 1 piece wholegrain toast with almond butter, or 1/2 tub of 0% plain Greek yogurt with honey, plus 1/2 cup of oats with honey and water.

Meal 2 (post workout): protein shake 60gms.

41

Meal 3 (lunch): 1 x chicken breast or 1 tin of tuna/fish 130gms with 1 x cup of spinach salad, 3 x tomatoes, 1/2 red onion, 5 x snap peas (no dressing), 1/2 cup brown rice or 1 x sweet potato.

Meal 4 (afternoon): homemade shake or 3 x rice cakes and almond butter.

Meal 5 (dinner): 1 x chicken or turkey breast or 1 x portion of fish (unprocessed) with 1 x cup of bean shoots, 1 x cup salad, 1 x cup spinach, and 1/4 cup of brown rice or 1 x sweet potato.

Meal 6 (evening): 1/2 cup of 0% cottage cheese with pepper or 1/2 cup of 0% plain Greek yogurt with honey and oats or protein shake 60gms.

Weeks 2-6

Meal 1 (breakfast): 5 egg whites + 1 yolk and 1 piece wholegrain toast with almond butter or 1/2 tub of 0% plain Greek yogurt with honey, plus 1/2 cup of oats with honey and water.

Post workout: protein shake 60gms.

Meal 2 (morning): turkey 150gms, brown rice 70gms and 2 x broccoli.

Meal 3 (lunch): 1 x chicken breast or 1 tin of tuna/fish 130gms, 1/2 cup brown rice or 1 x sweet potato.

Meal 4 (afternoon): homemade shake or 3 x rice cakes and almond butter.

Meal 5 (dinner): 1 x chicken or turkey breast or 1 x portion of fish (unprocessed) with 1 x cup of bean shoots, 1 x cup salad, 1 x cup spinach, and 1/4 cup of brown rice or 1 x sweet potato.

Meal 6 (evening): turkey 150gms, brown rice 70gms and 2 x broccoli.

Weeks 7-8

Meal 1 (breakfast): 1/2 cup of oats with honey and water.
Post workout: protein shake 60gms.

Meal 2 (morning): turkey 150gms, brown rice 70gms and 2 x broccoli.

Meal 3 (lunch): 1 x chicken breast or 1 tin of tuna/fish 130gms, 1/2 cup brown rice.

Meal 4 (afternoon): 3 x rice cakes

Meal 5 (dinner): 1 x chicken or turkey breast or 1 x portion of fish (unprocessed) with 1 x cup salad, 1 x cup spinach, and 1/4 cup of brown rice

Meal 6 (evening): turkey 150gms, brown rice 70gms and 2 x broccoli.

Weeks 9-12

Meal 1 (breakfast): 1/2 cup of oats with water.

Meals 2, 3, 4: turkey 150gms, brown rice 70gms and 2 x broccoli. (Post workout: protein shake 60gms)

Meals 5, 6: turkey 150gms, 8 x almonds and 2 x broccoli.

Photo-shoot Week

Meal 1 (breakfast): 1/2 cup of oats with water.

Meal 2, 3, 4, 5: turkey 150gms, 8 x almonds.

Fluids:

☐ Bottled mineral water – at least 4 litres per day plus water while training.

☐ Teas – unlimited natural teas with no added flavouring or chemicals. Try adding a tea bag to your bottled water to make a refreshing squash.

☐ Coffee – no more than one cup of black coffee per day. Avoid instant coffees and explore the different varieties of organic filter coffees instead.

Extras:

Daily

1 x daily multi-vitamin tablet
1 x post workout protein shake
2 x omega oil tablets
4 x BCAA tablets
1 x daily black coffee
1 x daily cube of dark chocolate (if needed)

Weekly

1 x weekly small glass of red wine or small bottle of ale
1 x weekly steak (red meat meal) as a Friday treat in lieu of dinner

Monthly

1 x monthly cheat meal – all to be consumed within 1 hour

AVOID!

The following are the items that should be removed from your diet from day one:

1. All dairy – this includes milk, cheese, or any substitutes except the whey protein ingredients.

2. Non-wholefoods – this includes anything refined, excluding the items listed within the meal plans.

3. Fruit – as you will see, fruit has not been listed in the meal plan, but it is included within the daily shakes.

4. Vegetables – stick to green vegetables such as broccoli and spinach

5. ALL PROCESSED FOODS

6. Sweeteners – this includes any sugars you may have added to your tea or coffee in the past.

Part Three
Training Schedule

This training schedule is divided into two sections.

1. Your daily schedule in the weights area: this part of the programme remains the same, so you will work the same sets of muscles on each day of the week for the next 12 weeks.

2. Your daily cardio schedule: this part of the programme changes every day throughout the 12 weeks and has been designed to gradually increase in intensity, thereby improving your overall cardiovascular fitness and fat burning ability.

Notes:

☐ The plan is to increase your weight-carrying capacity every 2 weeks, if not before.
☐ Super sets will be added from week 8 to add variety.
☐ Take a photo each Monday to keep a record of the physical changes; add this image to
your timeline at the rear of the book.
☐ Consume only water while training and add a protein-rich shake post workout.
☐ If possible, shower at the gym and look to socialise whenever possible with other
equally motivated individuals.
☐ Spend time looking at and appreciating your improvements in the mirror.

It is recommended to begin with the cardio aspect of the daily programme each time before hitting the weights. The cardio works as an ideal warm up, but remember that the cool down after your last set is of equal importance. Aim to work through a 5-minute routine of cool down stretches.

Here is an example of how to use the following:

Bench Press 15, 6, 8

Bench Press describes the exercise you will be performing, and **15, 6, 8** indicates that you will be completing three sets. The first set consists of 15 repetitions (lifts), the second set consists of 6 repetitions, and the third set consists of 8 repetitions.

Super Sets (beginning in week 8) – the term "super sets" describes a training routine in which you combine a number of different exercises and complete them one after the other. For example, in the routine listed below, your first set would be the exercises and repetitions highlighted in BOLD, the second set would be those highlighted in Italic, and the third set would be those highlighted Underlined .

Bench Press	**15,** *6,* <u>8</u>
Incline Bench	15, 10, 8, 6
Pullovers	**3,** *8,* <u>8,</u> 12
Pulldowns	**12,** *12,* <u>12</u>

The above exercises are performed one directly after the other with a rest time of 45 seconds between sets.

Daily Weights Workout

Monday:

Bench Press	**15,** *6,* <u>8</u>
Incline Bench	15, 10, 8, 6
Pullovers	**3,** *8,* <u>8,</u> 12
Pulldowns	**12,** *12,* <u>12</u>

Superset Squats	12, 12, 12
Crunches	15, 15, 15
Pull Ups	10, 10, 10
Push Ups	10, 10, 15
Sit Ups	15, 15, 15
Rope Seated Pull	10, 10, 10
Leg Raises	5, 5, 5

Tuesday:

Side Laterials	**12,** *12,* <u>12</u>
Upright Row	10, 10
Barbell Curl	**15,** *8,* <u>8</u>
Alternate Dumbell	**12,** *12,* <u>12</u>
Tricep Extentions	15, 10, 8, 6
Tricep Pushdowns	8, 10, 12
Pull Ups	10, 10, 10
Push Ups	10, 10, 15
Sit Ups	15, 15, 15
Rope Seated Pull	10, 10, 10

Wednesday:

Squats	**15,** *10,* <u>8,</u> 8
Front Squats	**3,** *5,* <u>8</u>
Leg Extentions	8, 8, 12
Lunges	8, 6, 10
Calf Raises	**6,** *8,* <u>8</u>
Pull Ups	10, 12, 12
Sit Ups	15, 15, 15
Rope Seated Pull	10, 15, 15

Thursday:

Incline Dumbell	**12,** *12,* <u>12</u>
Pullover	8, 10, 12
T-Bar Pulldown	**15,** *10,* <u>8,</u> 8
Reverse Grip Pull	**8,** *10,* <u>12</u>
Deadlift	8, 8, 12
Sit Ups	10, 15, 10
Push Ups	15, 15, 15
Pull Ups	10, 6, 8
Rope Seated Pull	10, 20, 20

Friday:

Seated Curls	**15,** *10,* <u>8</u>, 8
Seated Cable Row	**10,** *8,* <u>12</u>
Seated Side Laterals	8, 8, 8, 12
Cable Curls	**12,** *12,* <u>12</u>
Dips	12, 12, 12
Calf Raises	10, 10, 10
Sit Ups	15, 5, 5
Seated Rope Pull	10, 20, 20

Weekly Cardio Schedule

Week One:

- Monday – 2.4km run, best effort
- Tuesday – 20 minute jog
- Wednesday – 20 minute jog
- Thursday – 30 minute jog
- Friday – 20 minute cross trainer
- Saturday - rest
- Sunday - rest

Week Two:

- Monday – 20 minute run, best effort
- Tuesday – 400 metre swim / 20 minute cross trainer
- Wednesday – 10 minute run
- Thursday – 20 minute run
- Friday – 20 minute cross trainer or step
- Saturday – rest
- Sunday - rest

Week Three:

- Monday – 30 minute run, best effort
- Tuesday – 20 minute cross trainer
- Wednesday – 10 minute run
- Thursday – 40 minute steady pace jog
- Friday – 400 metre swim or 10 minute cross trainer
- Saturday - rest
- Sunday - rest

Week Four:

- Monday – 20 minute run, best effort
- Tuesday – 20 minute cross trainer
- Wednesday – 30 minute stead pace run
- Thursday – 10 minute row
- Friday – 400 metre swim or 20 minute cross trainer
- Saturday - rest
- Sunday - rest

Week Five:

- Monday – 2.4km run, best effort
- Tuesday – 20 minute swim or 10 minute cross trainer
- Wednesday – 20 minute cross trainer or step
- Thursday – 30 minute light jog

- Friday – 5 minute row, best effort
- Saturday - rest
- Sunday - rest

Week Six:

- Monday – 20 minute run
- Tuesday – 20 minute cross trainer
- Wednesday - 10 minute row
- Thursday – 20 minute swim or cross trainer
- Friday – 30 minute jog steady pace
- Saturday – rest or swim
- Sunday – rest or swim

Week Seven:

- Monday – 10 minute jog
- Tuesday – 20 minute cross trainer
- Wednesday – 15 minute run best effort
- Thursday – 10 minute row
- Friday – 20 minute swim or cross trainer
- Saturday – rest
- Sunday - rest

Week Eight:

- Monday – 30 minute run
- Tuesday – 400 meter swim or 20 minute cross trainer
- Wednesday – 15 minute row
- Thursday – rest
- Friday – 20 minute cross trainer
- Saturday - rest
- Sunday – 2hr hill walk

Week Nine:

- Monday – 10 minute swim
- Tuesday – 2.4km run best effort
- Wednesday – 10 minute row
- Thursday – 2 minute cross, 2 minute run, 2 minute bike
- Friday – rest or swim
- Saturday - rest
- Sunday – 1hr hill walk

Week Ten:

- Monday – 20 minute cross trainer
- Tuesday – 400 metre swim or 10 minute row
- Wednesday – 15 minute run
- Thursday – 5 minute cross, 5 minute run, 5 minute bike
- Friday – 20 minute cross trainer
- Saturday – rest or swim
- Sunday – rest or swim

Week Eleven:

- Monday – 30 minute run
- Tuesday – 5 minute cross, 5 minute run, 5 minute bike
- Wednesday – 10 minute row
- Thursday - rest
- Friday – 2.4km run, best effort
- Saturday – rest or swim
- Sunday – rest or 2hr hill walk

Week Twelve:

- Monday – 10 minute row
- Tuesday – 5 minute cross, 5 minute run, 5 minute bike
- Wednesday - 7 minute cross, 7 minute run, 7 minute bike
- Thursday - 5 minute cross, 5 minute run, 5 minute bike
- Friday - 7 minute cross, 7 minute run, 7 minute bike
- Saturday – rest or swim

•　　　Sunday – 20 minute swim or 2hr hill walk

Photoshoot Week:

Monday - 7 minute cross, 7 minute run, 7 minute bike
Tuesday - 5 minute cross, 5 minute run, 5 minute bike
Wednesday - 5 minute cross, 5 minute run, 5 minute bike
Thursday - rest
Friday – Photo-shoot

And this concludes the training programme. It goes without saying that much more can be learned on a deeper biological level, but the purpose of this book is not to delve too deep but rather to explore what you can do easily and effectively to bring lasting results.

As mentioned at the beginning of the book, if you wish to explore the science behind this programme's effectiveness in more detail, there are plenty of fantastic manuals and medical journals available in your local library.

Good luck. And remember, once you have committed, ensure you *complete* the programme.

Hard fact # 6: only 10 per cent of success is effort, the other 90 per cent is turning up!

Signing out ...

Benjamin

Your Photo Gallery

Within this area, why not take a picture, print it off and add it to your timeline....

Shopping List Week One

It's good practice to write out and record what quantities of food you are using on a weekly basis. Write out here what you have purchased within this period, this will enable you to plan for the following weeks.

Shopping List Week Two/Three/ Four/Five/Six

Shopping List Week Seven/ Eight

Shopping List Week Nine/Ten/ Eleven/Twelve

Shopping List Week Photoshoot/ Beach/Other

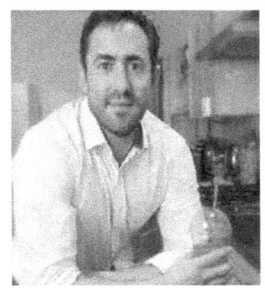

About Benjamin Bonetti

Using the three pillars of success, Benjamin Bonetti helps people become a better version of themselves. Through fitness, improving your mindset and well-being, and nutrition we can help you on your path to change. Having started out with a personal development company Empower Your Life in 2008, Benjamin Bonetti has gone on to become an established figure within the self-help sector.

Now one of the world's bestselling hypnotherapists and self-help authors, he has sold over 1 million self-help products across the world and regularly features in the top ten audio charts on Amazon, iTunes, Audible and the App Store. 2013 marks the relaunch of Benjamin Bonetti as a complete body and mind toolset, encompassing fitness plans, well-being programmes and nutritional supplements.

Having left school at 16, Benjamin served four years with the Royal Engineers travelling across the globe. He left the Army in 2003, ready to pursue his dream of owning his own business. Following a few false starts, he settled down to work at a local estate agency and went on to run his own independent estate agents, based in Worthing, West Sussex, which he sold in 2008.

It was at a NLP (Neuro-linguistic programming) course in 2008 that he met the MD of NLP World, Terry Elston. Following the course Benjamin became heavily involved with NLP, leading courses and working alongside Terry himself before establishing personal development company, Empower Your Life.

Team Bonetti Supporting Benjamin every step of the way, Team Bonetti work closely together to deliver exceptional service to Benjamin's clients. The Web, PR and Support teams, and Benjamin's management teams form the foundations of Team Bonetti. Benjamin Bonetti also sponsors a team of models and athletes, demonstrating what an individual can achieve - not only in their fitness, but also in their well-being and health.

Sponsored by:

WWW.BENJAMINBONETTI.COM

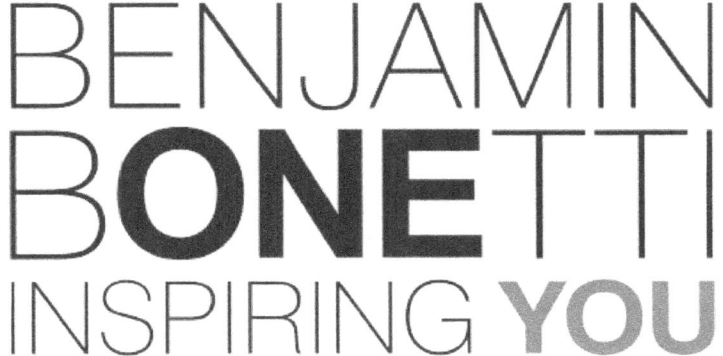

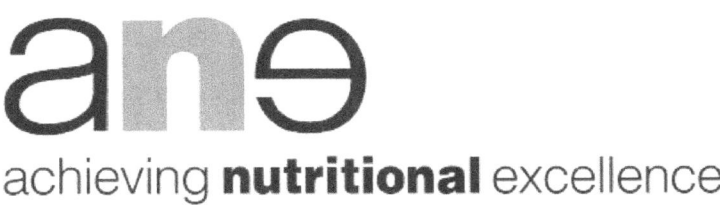